better nutrition *magazine* presents

CLEAR SKIN

by MYRA MICHELLE EBY

better nutrition
healthy living guide

Published by:
Active Interest Media, Inc.
300 N. Continental Blvd., Suite 650
El Segundo, CA 90245

This booklet is part of the *Better Nutrition Healthy Living Guide* series. For more information, visit www.betternutrition.com. Better Nutrition magazine is available at fine natural health stores throughout the United States. Design by Aline Design: Bellingham, Wash.

CLEAR SKIN

CONTENTS

better nutrition healthy living guide

Introduction

My Battle With Acne

I have battled acne and I know how it feels to look in the mirror when your complexion seems to be your worst enemy. It is difficult to think back to that time in my life when I was battling my acne, feeling frustrated and self-conscious.

My first blemish showed up shortly after I entered puberty, but unfortunately, it didn't just stop at one. My teen years were riddled with frequent breakouts. I endured hurtful, stereotypical name-calling and ridicule from my peers. Feeling unattractive and unsightly, I frequently shied away from cameras and smiles from strangers. But these skin problems were nothing compared to what lay ahead. Like a dark cloud, acne would follow me for years.

In my 20s, just when I thought I should be outgrowing my skin problems, my blemishes transformed into more severe cystic acne. At that time in my life, I quickly learned that one does not always just outgrow acne and that many other people were also affected with adult cystic acne. Unfortunately, my bout with acne lasted until my mid-30s.

Throughout the years, I spent many hours lamenting about my problem skin and tried every treatment and product I could get my hands on. Never seeing any lasting improvement, I grew increasingly frustrated by my condition. This frustration (and I know other acne-sufferers often feel the same way) was my biggest motivation to find a healthy solution to acne.

Vowing to find a solution and gain balanced, acne-free skin, I started with fasting and detoxification programs in addition to my already healthy diet. But because a healthy lifestyle is only part of the solution, I didn't experience any improvement. Since the hundreds of products I had tried didn't resolve the problem either, I finally decided to make my own skin care potions—more out of sheer desperation than anything else.

I scoured the bookshelves of local health food stores and found a fantastic book called *Jeanne Rose's Kitchen Cosmetics*. Imagine my surprise when I found recipes for problem skin that included fresh fruits, yogurt, and honey. Finally, I felt there was hope because I am a true believer in healing with foods. Because these skin care "smoothies" had such a beneficial effect on my skin, I began to experiment with a variety of fresh, natural ingredients that calmed my inflamed, blemished skin. The only problem—I had to make them fresh every day. I was also limited to what I could find at the grocery store.

Although my skin did improve with these homemade products, they didn't totally resolve my acne. I knew I was missing something—safe and natural bioactives to treat the underlying cause of my blemishes. I also knew I wasn't alone. Millions of people have spent years looking for a way to resolve their own skin problems, without success. That's when I decided to create MyChelle Dermaceuticals in 2000 and develop a series of products that combine the best nature and science have to offer, to help women reclaim healthy, glowing skin. Now, as my nieces and nephews are in the same boat as I was, I've focused on a series of effective, pure products that specifically target teenage acne.

But even the most effective products are only part of solving the acne puzzle. It's also important to understand how your skin works, the right way to care for it, and lifestyle changes that support a beautifully clear complexion. By practicing the skin care habits you'll learn about in this booklet, you will complete the puzzle and begin to see just how beautiful you really are.

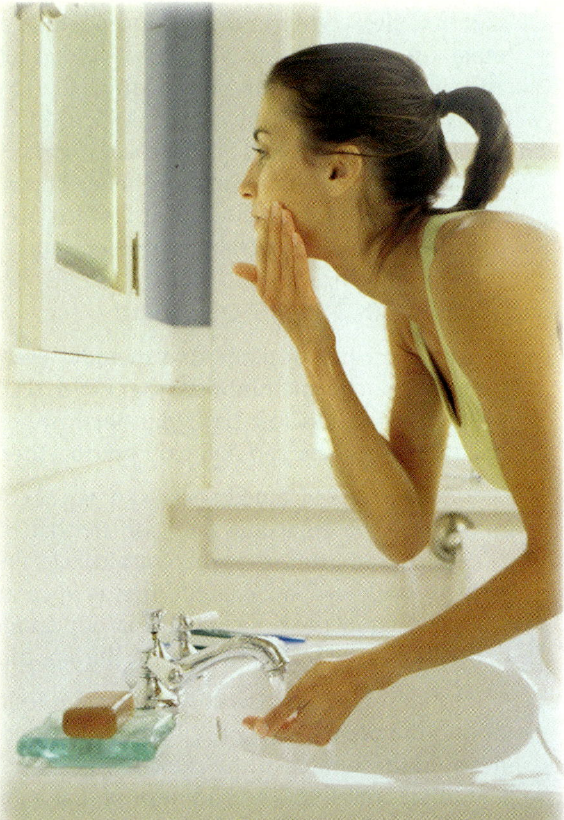

Millions of people have spent years looking for a way to resolve their own skin problems, without success.

Chapter One

The Challenge With Problem Skin

Acne can make you feel isolated, unattractive, and unlike anyone else you know. But the truth is, nearly 85 percent of people between the ages of 12 and 24 suffer from some type of acne—making it the most common type of skin disease on the planet. Of course, these statistics aren't going to clear up your skin or make you feel better. But knowing what you are up against can help you win the war against acne.

An acne lesion starts with increased oil production and a blockage in the hair follicles—pores in the skin from which a hair grows. The blockage is made up of sebum (an oily substance that lubricates your hair and skin) and dead skin cells; this combination literally plugs the pore and shows up as a whitehead or blackhead. When this condition occurs, bacteria—specifically, a type called *Propioni bacterium* or "P" bacteria—can then cause the infection and inflammation better known as pimples, blemishes, or zits. And these outbreaks aren't just limited to your face. They can also crop up on your neck, chest, back, shoulders, and even your upper arms.

The Five Types of Acne

Acne is a catchall name that includes everything from the occasional pimple to a chronic outbreak that never seems to go away. But all acne isn't the same. Doctors have identified five distinct types—and knowing what type you have can help you put together a good plan of attack.

Comedo Acne: Comedo—also known as comedones when there's more than one—is a sebaceous (oil) follicle that is plugged with sebum, dead skin cells from inside the sebaceous follicle, tiny hairs, and sometimes bacteria. A blackhead is a comedo that is open and exposed to the air, making the plug in the follicle black in appearance. A whitehead is a closed comedo covered by skin that looks like an inflamed "bump" on the skin.

Papule Acne: A papule is a small, solid lesion caused by a cellular reaction to the process of acne. The result is a slightly elevated bump with no head on the surface of the skin. The good news is that papule acne may be almost invisible. The bad news is that a group of these blemishes can make your skin feel like sandpaper.

Pustule Acne: A pustule is similar to a whitehead but is inflamed and appears as a red circle with a white or yellow center. Pustules are your garden-variety zit and consist of white blood cells, dead skin cells, and P. bacteria, which combine to create pus. If a pustule forms in a sebaceous follicle, it usually has a hair in the center.

Nodule Acne: This is a severe type of acne that can sometimes last for months and scarring is common. Nodules are large, hard bumps under the skin's surface that can be quite painful and may cause tissue destruction in the deeper layers of the skin. Unresolved nodules can sometimes leave an impaction behind, which can flare again and again.

Cyst Acne: Another severe form of acne, cyst acne can look a little like a nodule, but it is filled with pus from white blood cells, dead skin cells, and bacteria. While that might sound like a pustule, it isn't. Instead, a cyst can be as big as 1/8-inch across and can be very painful. Like nodule acne, cyst acne often results in scarring. Making matters worse, cysts and nodules can occur together in a really severe form of acne called nodulocystic acne that is likely to leave scars once it has healed.

What's Causing Acne?

Nobody really knows why some people get acne and others don't. But there are some risk factors that seem to contribute to its development. Family history is one. While you can't blame your family for all the problems in your life, if either of your parents suffered from acne, you are more likely to develop it, too—and earlier than if you didn't have a family history of the condition.

But even if your parents suffered only the occasional zit, don't think you are home-free. Hormonal changes in your body can trigger or aggravate acne. During puberty, you go through a number of changes as your body begins to produce hormones called androgens. Unfortunately, an increase in androgen levels causes the sebaceous glands to get larger. Higher levels of these hormones also cause the skin to make more sebum. As the sebum travels up the follicle toward the surface of the skin, it mixes with dead skin cells and bacteria, increasing the chances of clogged pores.

All teens are prone to breakouts. Girls often experience more sporadic flare-ups because they have fluctuating hormone levels during their menstrual cycle. Girls can also experience an outbreak because of the cosmetics they use. But boys are more likely than girls to experience more severe, longer lasting forms of acne.

People with chronic or more severe forms of acne may also suffer from sluggish skin cell turnover. Normally, the rate of healthy skin cell turnover is every 21 to 28 days. That means that about once a month, the dead cells inside the follicles rise to the surface of the skin, where they are removed through washing and other everyday activities.

And then there are bacteria. Your skin is home to millions of bacteria—some good, some bad. P. bacteria is a bad bacteria and is the culprit behind infectious acne. If a follicle becomes plugged and oil glands are actively pumping out oil, this bacteria multiplies rapidly, causing red, painful inflammation.

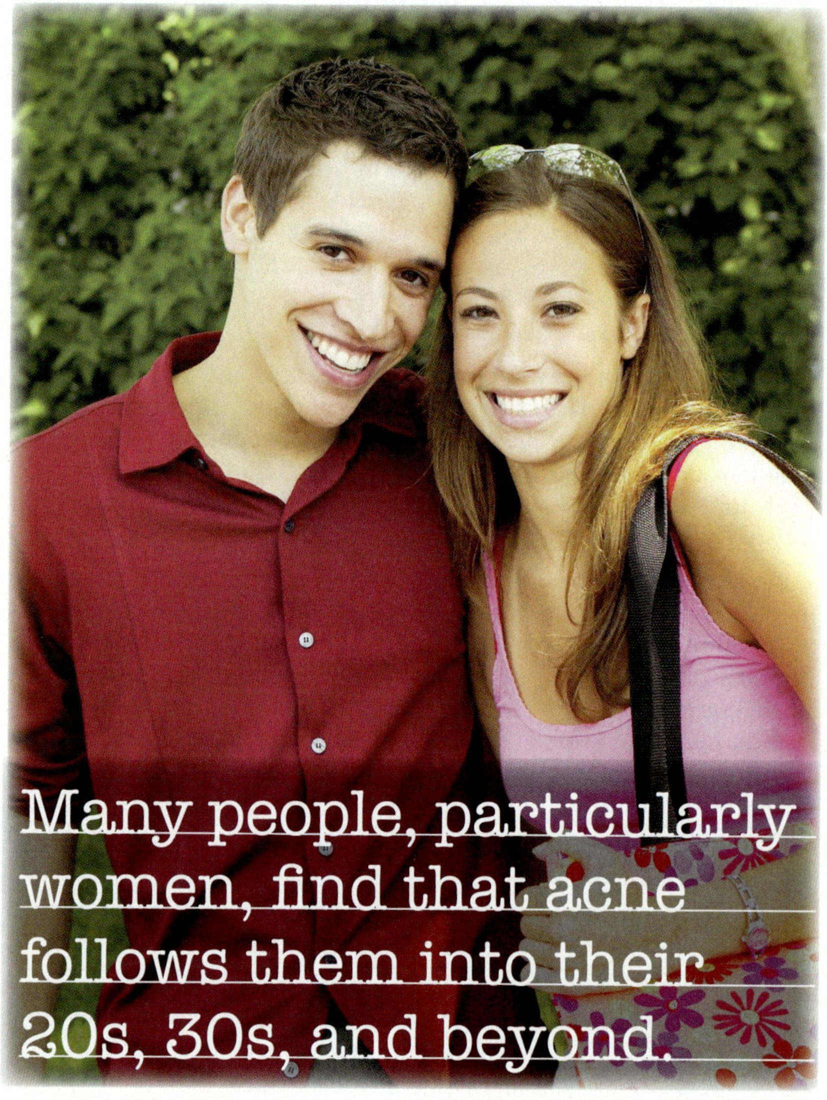

Now that you understand acne a little better, let's talk about some acne myths you might have heard:

Myth No. 1: Acne is caused by poor hygiene. This myth probably comes from the fact that blackheads look like dirt that's stuck in your pores, which they actually are. But poor hygiene is not what initiates the formation of acne deep in the hair follicle. Gentle and regular exfoliation will minimize and reduce blackhead-prone skin.

Myth No. 2: Acne is just a cosmetic disease. Yes, acne does affect the way people look and is not otherwise a serious threat to a person's physical health. However, acne can result in permanent physical scars. Plus, acne itself, as well as its scars, can negatively affect the way people feel about themselves to the point of affecting their lives.

Myth No. 3: You'll outgrow your acne. Yes, some people do find that as they leave their teen years, their skin clears up. But many people, particularly women, find that acne follows them into their 20s, 30s, and beyond. Waiting for your acne to "go away" without treating it properly can lead to frequent breakouts, scarring, and a lack of self-esteem.

Myth No. 4: The sun will help get rid of your acne. Getting a tan—or worse, a sunburn—can seem to make your acne less visible. But UV exposure causes irritation, which can make acne worse. What's more, the sun's rays can damage the newly formed skin that results from an effective acne treatment. Too much sun also damages your skin, which can accelerate skin aging and increase your risk of skin cancer.

Myth No. 5: Sweating cleans out your pores. While exercise is an important part of a healthy lifestyle, it can cause flare-ups for some people. Vigorous exercise stimulates oil production, which, when combined with heat, perspiration, and friction, aggravates acne on the forehead, chest, and back. You can minimize irritation by wearing loose cotton clothing and by showering immediately after exercising.

Myth No. 6: Popping pimples will help them go away faster. Even though extracting a pimple may make it temporarily seem less noticeable, it can cause the blemish to stick around longer. Improperly extracting clogged pores or inflamed lesions can push bacteria farther into the skin while making the area around the acne even more reddened and inflamed. Extracting devices—such as "blackhead extractors" advertised in magazines—aren't any safer. Sometimes improper extraction can cause red scars to form that could last months; and scarring, in the form of dents and pits, can last forever.

Myth No. 7: Acne is contagious. This popular myth is spread mostly by fathers to keep their teenage girls away from acne-covered boys! Nothing you do will either cause you to "catch" acne or "give" it to someone else.

Chapter Two
Conventional Wisdom?

If you are looking for something that claims to magically make your acne go away, you don't have to look far. Drugstore shelves are packed with dozens of creams and potions that promise clear skin—and you've probably tried many of them, without success. Dermatologists, armed with industrial-strength drugs, offer even more promises—some that may even work temporarily. But most people aren't aware of the long list of nasty side effects that come with these promises.

Drugstore Pipe Dreams

Cosmetic counters are littered with medicated creams or pads designed to help control mild to moderate acne. But many of these products contain harsh chemicals that can actually make the problem worse by drying out and irritating your skin.

Benzoyl peroxide is the most common ingredient in over-the-counter zit zappers like Clinque Acne Solutions, ProActiv, and ZAPZYT Acne Treatment Gel. Benzoyl peroxide is a drying and bleaching agent that works by killing the P. bacteria. It also helps unclog pores and reduces inflammation of the skin. Most over-the-counter treatments contain 2.5 percent benzoyl peroxide, but some products are packed with up to 10 percent.

Side effects are dose-dependent, which means that the higher the concentration, the more likely it is you will suffer adverse effects—including excessive dryness and flaking, redness, peeling, and burning. More seriously, studies show that benzoyl peroxide also damages DNA—molecules in the body that contain your genetic information. Although the Food and Drug Administration (FDA) and the cosmetic industry claim that benzoyl peroxide is safe, the Environmental Working Group classifies it as a hazardous chemical. It is also listed on Canada's "Hot List" of ingredients that aren't allowed in products sold in that country.

Another antibacterial agent used in acne products is triclosan, a broad-spectrum antibacterial found in Clearasil, Phisoderm, and Noxema. It is especially effective against P. bacteria, but the Environmental Protection Agency classifies triclosan as a pesticide and as a risk to both human health and the environment. Swedish studies have found high levels of triclosan in the blood and breast milk of women using personal care products containing the chemical, which means that triclosan does get absorbed into the body. Other research shows that it is stored in the body's fatty tissue, where it can hang around for decades. Always check ingredient labels, and avoid any product containing triclosan.

Dermatology's Dark Side

People who suffer from moderate to severe acne rarely get much relief from over-the-counter products. Instead, many turn to a dermatologist in a desperate attempt to resolve their skin problems. Yet exposure to the strong treatments dermatologists often use can leave your skin in worse shape than when you made the first appointment. I have talked with many people who have been scarred for life by a doctor trying to "fix" the problem. Others have ended up battling long-term physical or psychological troubles after taking prescription acne drugs.

Antibiotics are one of the most popular ways dermatologists treat stubborn acne, and they can be used both topically and internally. Antibiotic treatments applied to the surface of the skin kill the bacteria hiding out in blocked follicles. The most popular topical antibiotic is Clindamycin. Because it attacks both gram-negative and gram-positive bacteria, it's an effective tool against both P. bacteria and any infection that can arise from acne. But slathering on a Clindamycin gel or foam isn't without risk.

Oral antibiotics used to treat acne include erythromycin or one of the tetracycline drugs. Essentially, these drugs also kill bacteria, but from the inside out. While dermatologists are quick to prescribe these drugs, reducing the P. bacteria will not, in itself, do anything to reduce the oil secretion and abnormal cell behavior that are the root causes of blocked follicles. Plus, the antibiotics used to treat acne are becoming less and less effective as the bacteria develop a resistance against the drugs. As a result, acne often reappears soon after the treatment has ended—days later, in the case of topical treatments, and weeks later, in the case of oral antibiotics.

One type of tetracycline, called minocycline, may have several worrisome side effects. Reports of hypersensitivity, liver problems, and drug-induced lupus have dermatologists thinking twice before prescribing this drug to their patients. Two patients have also died after taking minocycline.

Antibiotics, especially when taken orally, can also cause other problems. Even if you only take them for a short time, these drugs upset the bacterial balance in your body by killing both the bad bacteria that contribute to your acne and beneficial bacteria. Low levels of these beneficial bugs have been linked to a number of common digestive disorders. They've also been implicated in jock itch and yeast infections. And surprisingly, some natural health practitioners suspect that waning levels of beneficial bacteria contribute to gingivitis, psoriasis, eczema, migraines, urinary tract infections, and chronic fatigue syndrome.

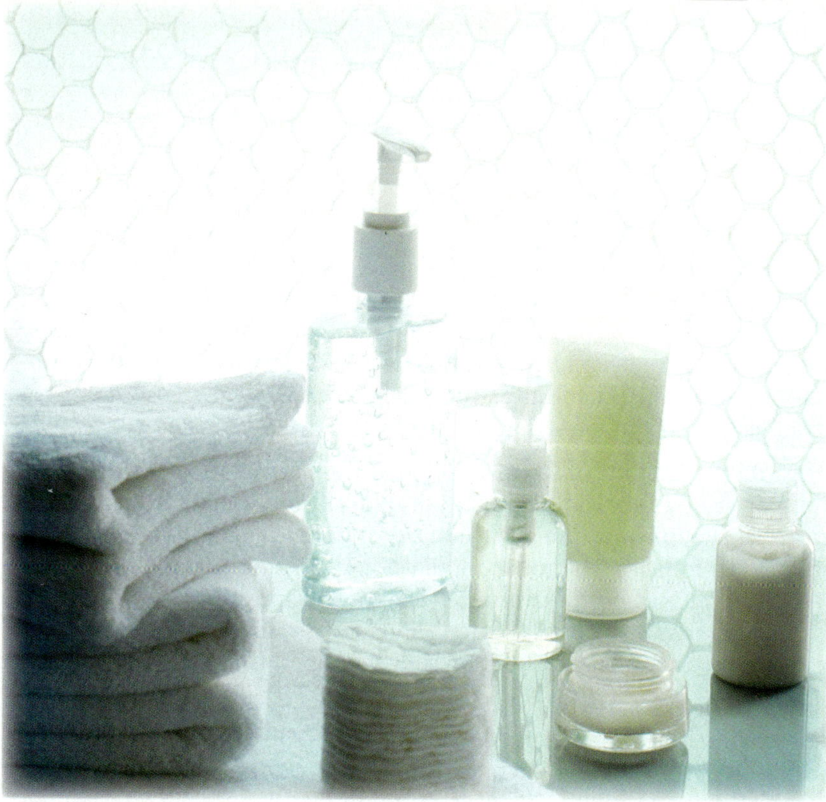

But antibiotics aren't the only medications dermatologists rely on. Topical retinoid drugs used to normalize the life cycle of follicle cells are also popular. These drugs, known as Retin-A, Differin, and Tazorac, are vitamin-A derivatives, so it sounds like they should be good for you. But before you get too excited, you need to know that these topical retinoids can cause significant skin irritation, as well as an initial flare-up of acne and facial flushing.

Skin to Die For: The Accutane Debate

Probably the most controversial acne drug is Accutane—technically known as isotretinoin. Like Retin-A, it's a cousin to vitamin A, but that's where the similarity ends. Accutane was originally used to treat severe, disfiguring cystic acne. It works by shrinking the oil glands and reducing the amount of oil your skin produces.

While the results from Accutane can be impressive, the side effects are numerous and widespread. They can include hair loss, vision problems, neurological symptoms (dizziness, drowsiness, seizures, and stroke), the rapid breakdown of muscles, joint and muscle pain, long-lasting arthritis, elevated liver enzymes, inflammatory bowel disease, an inflamed pancreas, and respiratory problems. Doctors warn women who take the drug not to become pregnant since Accutane causes devastating birth defects. The risks of Accutane on unborn children is so severe that female patients are required to use two forms of birth control while on the drug—whether they are sexually active or not.

But the side effect that has really grabbed headlines is Accutane's link to depression and suicide. Shortly after Accutane became legal in 1982, patients began to report depressive symptoms while taking the drug, leading the drug's maker—Roche Laboratories—to put the following label on the package: "WARNING: Accutane may cause depression, psychosis and, rarely, suicidal ideation, suicide attempts and suicide." But it wasn't until the year 2000, when Michigan congressman Bart Stupak's son BJ committed suicide while on the drug, that Accutane's deadly potential came to light. Yet, even though many studies were conducted, there wasn't any conclusive evidence tying the acne drug to an uptick in depression—that is, not until a 2006 study showed depression-related behavior in mice injected with the drug. This was followed up by a large human crossover study in 2008 clearly linking Accutane, suicide, and depression.

Even with all of these life-altering (and potentially deadly) side effects, Accutane is overprescribed. Most experts agree that Accutane should be reserved for people with extremely severe cystic acne who do not respond to other treatments. Personally, I don't think that Accutane should ever be given to patients. Acne may be discomforting, even debilitating, but so many of these Accutane side effects can be truly tragic.

Birth Control For Better Skin?

For years doctors have used oral contraceptives as off-label acne treatments for women. Today, a handful of oral contraceptives are also FDA-approved as acne treatments. Since birth control pills reduce the amount of testosterone within the body, they often improve hormonally based acne breakouts. When testosterone production is suppressed, it reduces the amount of oil produced by the sebaceous glands. The chance of pore blockages is also reduced.

But taking "the pill" isn't without risk. You can experience nausea, weight gain, breast tenderness, menstrual spotting and mood swings. More serious problems can also occur, such as blood clots, stroke, gallstones, an increase in blood pressure and depression. Using birth control pills to prevent pregnancy is a personal choice, but there are safer, more natural ways to treat your acne.

Chapter Three
Heal Acne Naturally

According to The Acne Resource Center, three out of every four teens experience acne. Twenty-five percent of them will be left with permanent scars. Because of my own battle with acne, I know how incredibly frustrating it can be to try countless treatments that don't work. Instead, you find that your skin is on a roller-coaster ride between excessive dryness and oil overload. But I can also tell you from personal experience that you can live an acne-free life by adopting a natural, pure approach to your complexion.

The chemically filled acne products you find in the drug or department store often swear that you'll see results within days or weeks. The creams and cleansers sold exclusively online often make even more outrageous claims. The truth is, healing takes time and proper care. Improvements won't appear in the mirror overnight, but you'll probably see a change for the better in a month or two—and if you continue the skin-smart strategies I've outlined in this chapter, your progress will prove long-lasting.

The Rules

Every little thing you do counts when it comes to fighting acne and keeping it under control. Even mindless habits—like scratching your face—can aggravate your skin. What you don't do is just as important as what you do. Avoiding behavior that irritates skin can also help keep your complexion clear.

DO clean your face twice a day, typically in the morning and again before bed. If you exercise or play sports, wash your face after your workout to get rid of sweat.

DO protect your skin from harsh environmental factors such as sun and wind since they can make your skin more vulnerable to infection.

DO shampoo your hair regularly. The oil glands on your scalp produce the same sebum that's on your face.

DO keep your hair pulled back off your face, and don't let hair products touch your skin.

DO choose noncomedogenic cosmetics that won't clog pores.

DO change your sheets often—especially pillowcases. Since your face rests on your pillowcase every day, the pillowcase absorbs the oil from your skin. A soiled pillowcase can redeposit dirt and oil.

DON'T use rough washcloths or loofahs on areas where acne is present.

DON'T scrub your face vigorously. A gentle touch is just as effective for ridding your skin of dirt and oil.

DON'T ever go to bed without first washing away dirt, oil and makeup.

DON'T rest your chin in your hands or touch your skin unless absolutely necessary.

DON'T hold your cell phone against your face.

DON'T squeeze or pop blemishes—ever! Yes, I know it's tempting, but squeezing can allow a secondary infection to take hold and may lead to permanent scarring.

Adopt a "Clear Skin" Routine

Rules are fine—and they can help manage your acne. But they are no substitute for a good skin care routine. Consistency is the key to controlling your acne. Acne can be very opportunistic, so hit-or-miss skin care can open the door to outbreaks. But it can be hard to stick with a skin care program if the only products available are so harsh that they irritate your skin or they don't live up to their claims. That was the problem I had growing up. And that's why I was compelled to develop a series of safe and effective acne products just for teens. The series, called Clear Skin Teen Anthology, is the first step toward an acne-free future, and it covers all the bases: cleansing, toning, targeting emerging and full-blown pimples and moisturizing.

Acne-free skin starts as clean skin. Cleansing removes dirt, dead skin cells and makeup. It also controls oil production, reduces bacteria and promotes normal cell turnover. But before you reach for that bar of soap, be aware that soaps are highly alkaline and can strip the skin of natural oils. Not only does removing all the sebum from your skin disrupt the natural lipid barrier, it can send oil production into overdrive in the body's effort to rebalance moisture levels. But even after sebum returns, the skin's barrier and bacterial balance remains compromised, notes Kat James, author of *The Truth About Beauty*. "As a result," she adds, "blemishes and other inflammatory problems are more likely to occur until the barrier is re-established."

Most mainstream antibacterial cleansers designed for acne also strip skin with harsh detergents like sodium lauryl sulfate or antibacterial ingredients like lauramidopropyl betaine. These petroleum-based chemicals can also irritate skin as they melt away dead skin cells and dislodge the dirt. Cleansers based on antibacterial botanicals, on the other hand, are created to kill the P. bacteria as they dissolve and wash away impurities—all without stripping the skin's natural oils. I've found one powerful herbal extract that is incredibly effective against the acne-causing bacteria on the surface of the skin. Totarol, which comes from the totara tree in New Zealand, is a thousand times more effective than tea tree oil against P. bacteria. Additionally, it is an exceptional antioxidant. Search for Totarol online to learn more about this amazing extract

But killing bacteria is only part of the battle. Your cleanser should also gently exfoliate your skin with a natural source of salicylic acid like willow bark. Willow bark not only delivers antibacterial properties, it also dissolves dead skin cells, which helps to prevent clogged pores.

Next comes toning. Ideally, toners should provide natural antioxidants and anti-inflammatory herbs to target acne while nourishing the skin. But many over-the-counter toners contain alcohol and acetone, which can be extremely drying for even the oiliest complexion. If you have very oily skin, drying it out might not sound like a bad idea. But overdrying your skin will pull debris even deeper into your pores, making it hard for your skin to naturally excrete the impurities that lead to blackheads and whiteheads.

Conventional toners can also include plasticizers like polyvinylpyrrolidone (PVP), which gives skin that "tight" feeling. This plastic resin can be absorbed by the skin and may remain in the body for months after use. You can also find synthetic colors, fragrances and preservatives in these products, making them potentially irritating to your skin. But there are safer and more soothing ways to tone your skin and target your acne.

Instead of alcohol or dubious chemicals, I've found that natural antimicrobials, such as supercritical extracted Totarol and neem, neutralize infection-causing bacteria like the P. bacteria without stripping the skin. I've combined these two exotic botanicals with lemongrass essential oil, red grapefruit essential oil and willow bark in my Clear Skin Clarifying Pads. Lemongrass essential oil is one of my favorites due to its calming effects on overactive sebaceous glands. Not only does it smell delicious and uplifting, but studies also show that it contains potent antioxidant properties, as well as the ability to soothe painful pimples and reduce swelling. As a result, these convenient pads attack bacteria, reduce pore size, encourage continued exfoliation and calm the skin.

If you suffer from more than the occasional blemish, applying a concentrated serum specifically formulated to reduce oil production, calm inflammation and reduce the risk of scarring can really benefit your skin. But be aware that many spot treatments contain benzoyl peroxide, alcohol and petroleum derivatives that can make matters worse by drying and irritating skin, leaving blemishes crusty and hard to conceal. Instead of targeting blemishes with toxins, a natural spot treatment uses concentrated amounts of pure ingredients proven to reduce acne. My Clear Skin

Most acne-prone skin actually suffers from a lack of hydration, which can also set up your complexion for premature aging.

Spot Treatement is specifically formulated for this type of intense blemish attack, relying on powerful Totarol extract combined with the antibacterial, antifungal power of sulfur. Sulfur is a natural element found in the earth's crust, and it can stimulate healing when used on damaged skin.

Moisturizing (nourishing) is the fourth step in my daily skin care plan. This may sound counterintuitive to those with oily skin, but lack of moisture can trigger inflammation and compromise the skin's ability to heal itself. Most acne-prone skin actually suffers from a lack of hydration, which can also set up your complexion for premature aging. As I developed my Clear Skin Balancing Moisturizer, I knew it was vital to provide moisture and minimize bacteria on the surface of the skin. It was also important to balance the skin's oil production without it becoming overly dry, since this would simply cause the skin to hyper-produce oil again.

Your skin loses moisture every day, and moisturizers are designed to counter this water loss. While natural moisturizers provide a bounty of botanical humectants, synthetic moisturizers are another story. Relying on mainstream moisturizers may actually sabotage your skin's moisture content. Instead of natural oils and plant-based emollients, most brand-name moisturizers are packed with petrochemicals such as mineral oil and petrolatum. These refined crude oil products lie on the surface of the skin, effectively preventing the skin's normal respiration. Since these compounds also clog pores, they can prevent the release of toxins and waste, resulting in blemish outbreaks. And although all moisturizers make our skin feel smooth and soft immediately after we apply them, these synthetic compounds may actually pull moisture from the skin.

To safely keep your skin hydrated, it's important to use a moisturizer containing natural humectants like vegetable glycerin—which pull moisture from the air and into your skin—as well as plant-based emollients like aloe vera that help seal in the water and condition the skin. Unlike synthetic moisturizers, these pure ingredients are noncomedogenic and won't block pores.

Because nourishing moisturizers are absorbed by the skin, they are the perfect vehicle for adding acne-specific herbs. Along with bacteria-blitzing supercritical extracted Totarol, I've found that daisy extract contains astringent and anti-inflammatory properties to calm redness and swelling. Daisy is also excellent for anyone suffering from acne scarring since it brightens scars, making them less visible.

Skin Treats

A regular skin care routine, practiced morning and night, will go a long way toward alleviating acne. But for anyone who suffers from more than the occasional pimple, more needs to be done. Gentle, consistent exfoliation is critical if you want to genuinely extinguish acne. Exfoliation removes the dead skin cells that contribute to blackheads. Even today, exfoliation is the key to keeping my acne under control. If I forget to exfoliate, my pores are more prone to becoming clogged, eventually leading to a blemish breakout.

In recent years, fruit enzymes have become a popular way to exfoliate the skin. These enzymes, found in fruits like pineapple and pumpkin, dissolve dead skin cells and support proper skin respiration. As a result, these gentle enzymatic exfoliators help unplug clogged pores by removing the loosened cells, which normally stick together on the skin's surface.

Mud masks are another wonderful way to detoxify pores and enhance cell turnover while providing antioxidants and healing minerals to the skin. My favorite mask, the Cranberry Mud Mask, is composed of bentonite and kaolin clays, which absorb oil and pull impurities from pores. Add to that, supercritical extracted Totarol to neutralize bacteria, green tea, rosemary essential oil and fruit extracts to reduce inflammation and free radicals, and herbs to nourish the skin.

Masks go on wet and work their magic as they dry on your skin. A unique feature of MyChelle's Cranberry Mud Mask is that it DOES NOT completely dry on the skin, as this would send your skin into yet another round of oil hyper-production. It's important to thoroughly remove all traces of the mask once it has dried—usually in 10 to 15 minutes—with a thoroughly moist, warm, clean washcloth in a gentle, circular motion. It is also important that you don't use a mud mask too often since this can irritate your skin. Once or twice a week should be enough to improve your skin, with the exception of daily spot treatments when necessary until the desired results are achieved. Follow with a toner and moisturizer.

Clear Skin For Teens

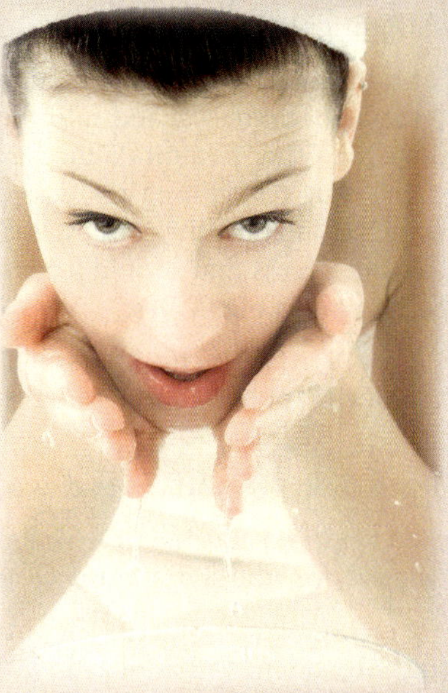

Four Steps to Acne-Free Skin

To have truly healthy skin, it's important to cleanse, tone, spot treat, and moisturize twice a day, every day, morning and evening. Following these four steps neutralizes the P. bacteria, normalizes oil production, and helps prevent impurities and dead skin cells from clogging your pores.

Clean: Gently massage a small amount of Clear Skin Cleanser into your face using small, circular motions. Rinse well with warm (not hot or cold) water to remove all traces of cleanser and dirt.

Tone: Follow your cleansing by gently wiping your face with a Clear Skin Clarifying Pad to fight bacteria, rebalance the skin's natural pH, and refine the pores while supporting the healing process of the skin. Always use a fresh pad, and never rub the pad across your skin since it may damage delicate tissue. If your skin is especially oily, or if your acne extends to your torso, use more than one pad as needed.

Treat: Dab a small amount of Clear Skin Spot Treatment onto active breakouts. This treatment can be used sparingly on one pimple, or try one to two pumps on a larger area if necessary. You will also notice that as the Clear Skin Spot Treatment dries, it also works as a great cover-up.

Moisturize: Apply Clear Skin Balancing Moisturizer immediately after cleansing and when skin is still slightly damp. Simply dab a bit of the oil-free moisturizer on your cheeks, chin, nose, and forehead, and gently massage it into your skin. Wait a few minutes for the moisturizer to be absorbed before applying makeup. (Please note that if you do not use makeup, you may add a little more Clear Skin Spot Treatment on inflamed areas to minimize the appearance of your blemishes.)

Acne-Fighting Ingredients

Mother Nature has given us all the tools we need for clear skin. Some of these, like tea tree oil and salicylic acid, are probably familiar to you. But there are other botanicals that are even more effective acne fighters. I've spent years researching and sourcing these ingredients from around the world to find only the gentlest, safest, and most effective of them. Here are the ingredients that should form the basis of your natural arsenal in your battle against blemishes:

Aloe Vera Gel: This hydrating, softening, and healing emollient from the aloe plant has antimicrobial and anti-inflammatory properties.

Bentonite Clay: A natural white clay that absorbs excess oil and pulls debris from pores when used as a mask.

Chamomile Extract: Skin-calming herb that rebalances dryness and helps restore the skin's radiance and freshness.

Cranberry Extract: This bright red berry nourishes skin while providing antioxidant and antibacterial activity.

Daisy Extract: Daisy has astringent and calming properties, and it is used to refresh the skin while helping to rebalance oiliness.

Fruit Enzymes: The protein-digesting enzymes in some types of fruit have the ability to digest dead skin cells on the surface of the skin, revealing a smooth, fresh appearance.

Glycerin (Vegetable): A natural humectant derived from palm kernel oil, glycerin is excellent for smoothing and moisturizing the skin. Specifically, glycerin helps to prevent moisture loss and skin dehydration.

Green Tea Extract: Rich in natural plant antioxidants, green tea helps maintain a smooth, balanced complexion by protecting the skin from damaging free radicals.

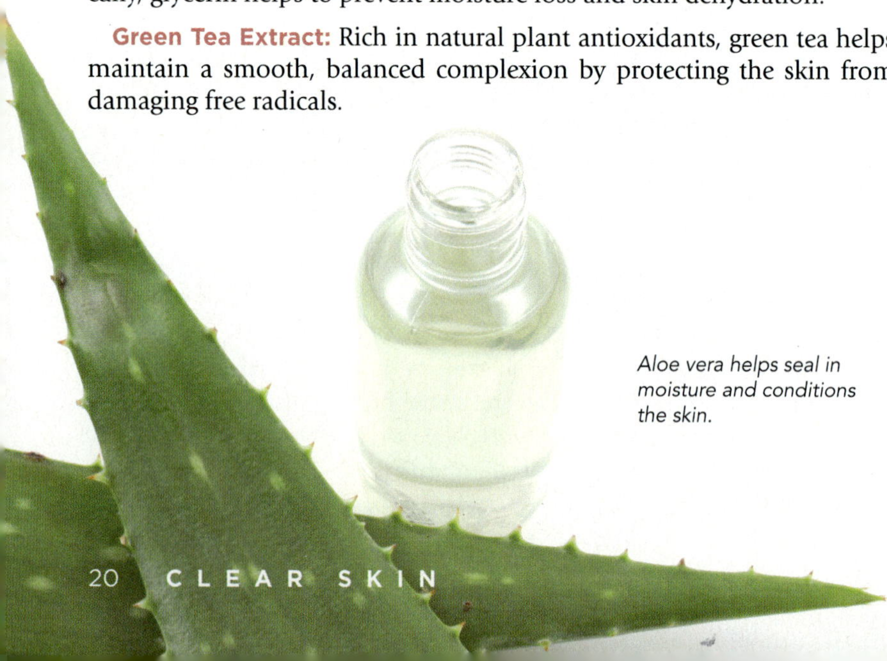

Aloe vera helps seal in moisture and conditions the skin.

Ingredients to Avoid

It's important to check the ingredient labels on all the products you use on your skin, including hair care products and color cosmetics. Avoid the ingredients listed below. Although a few come from plants, most are derived from petroleum and can either clog your pores or irritate acne-prone skin. Some are also toxic and can cause cancer, disrupt hormones, or trigger an allergic reaction.

- Acetone
- Butyl stearate
- Cinnamon oil
- Cocoa butter (Avoid highly refined product only)
- Coconut oil (Avoid highly refined product only)
- Decyl oleate
- Isocetyl stearate
- Isopropyl isostearate
- Isopropyl myristate
- Isopropyl palmitate
- Isostearyl isostearate
- Isostearyl neopentanoate
- Lanolin
- Mineral oil
- Myristyl myristate
- Myristyl propionate
- Octyl palmitate
- Octyl stearate
- Petrolatum
- Sodium lauryl/laureth sulfates

Kaolin Clay: Kaolin is a naturally sourced clay that helps to rebalance oiliness and absorb impurities. It contains beneficial minerals and trace elements that help leave skin feeling hydrated and refreshed.

Neem: Studies show that the oil from this native Indian tree has exceptionally strong antibacterial, antifungal, and antiseptic properties that benefit acne and help preserve the skin's elasticity.

Pineapple Enzymes: Derived from the stems of pineapple, these enzymes exfoliate skin by digesting dead cells. As a result, pineapple enzymes have a skin-softening effect.

Plantago: Used since prehistoric times to soothe skin abrasions, this plant has anti-inflammatory, astringent, and antimicrobial properties.

Pumpkin Enzymes: Pumpkin is a rich source of antioxidants and enzymes that act like alpha-hydroxy acids. Pumpkin also contains more than 100 beneficial nutrients that can help reverse the signs of aging.

Rooibos Tea Extract: Japanese scientists found that rooibos tea contains a compound that mimics superoxide dismutase (SOD), an antioxidant that attacks free radicals and limits their damaging effects on the skin.

Rosemary: Rosemary contains potent antioxidants and a natural compound called ursolic acid, which has skin restorative properties. Rosemary invigorates and enlivens the skin and scalp, rebalancing oiliness.

Salicylic Acid: This compound occurs naturally in wintergreen and willow bark. Salicylic acid effectively helps the skin shed dead cells, even at low concentrations. It also has antiseptic properties.

Seabuckthorn Extract: Packed with nutrients, seabuckthorn contains high levels of vitamins C, E, K, B1, B2, and A, along with beta-carotene, lycopene, zeaxanthin, and fatty acids. Studies show that when used this topically, this nutritional powerhouse helps heal wounds.

Tea Tree Oil: This Australian essential oil has long been used as a natural antiseptic and antibacterial, as well as a cleansing agent that rebalances oiliness.

Totarol: A naturally occurring supercritical extracted plant extract from New Zealand with potent antibacterial and antioxidant properties. It's 1,000 times more potent than tea tree oil against the P. bacteria.

Willow Bark: A natural source of salicylic acid that helps enhance cell turnover by exfoliating the skin. It effectively and gently dissolves dirt and impurities that may clog pores.

Witch Hazel: A refreshing astringent, with clarifying and toning properties. It helps to reduce oiliness while calming and smoothing the skin.

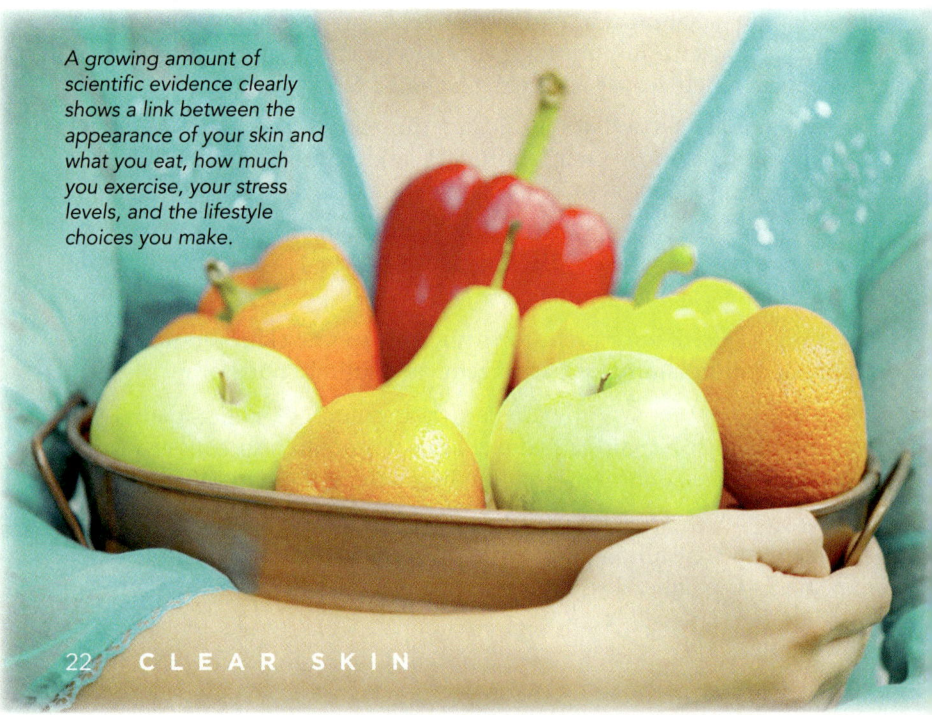

A growing amount of scientific evidence clearly shows a link between the appearance of your skin and what you eat, how much you exercise, your stress levels, and the lifestyle choices you make.

Chapter Four
Healthy Skin Habits

As important as it is to use effective, pure products on your skin, a clear complexion isn't just skin deep. Your skin is a mirror of your overall health—and that begins on the inside.

A growing amount of scientific evidence clearly shows a link between the appearance of your skin and what you eat, how much you exercise, your stress levels, and the lifestyle choices you make. Yes, we all know people with flawless skin who live on junk food, sit in front of the TV for hours on end, and generally abuse their bodies. Trust me, their bad habits will catch up with them sooner or later. But if you suffer from acne, these bad habits can make your condition worse—no matter what topical treatments you use. Choosing healthy habits, on the other hand, supports the outer efforts you make and will reward you with clearer skin, proper digestion, a stronger immune system, and energy to spare.

Diet

According to the Chinese, a healthy diet is a key factor in maintaining a healthy complexion. Traditional Chinese medicine sees the skin as the body's secondary elimination organ. When the flow of "chi" (vital energy) to the liver and colon is blocked, the body releases fats and toxins through the skin, often resulting in blemishes. The traditional Chinese diet supports this philosophy, relying on organically fermented soy products, fresh fruits and vegetables, and grains to maintain flawless skin.

The typical American diet, however, is full of highly processed foods, artery-clogging animal fat, and refined sugars and starches. Recent research shows that eliminating junk food from your diet results in a clearer complexion, debunking the widespread belief that food plays no role in the development of acne. A study published in the *American Journal of Clinical Nutrition* shows a link between high-glycemic foods (those high in sugar and processed grains) and acne. When a group of young men, ages 15 to 25, abandoned their typical diet of overly processed and high-sugar foods for 12 weeks of healthy eating (whole grains, lean meat and fish, and fruits and vegetables), their acne decreased by 51 percent.

Researchers believe that foods high on the glycemic index cause blood sugar to spike. The body reacts by releasing a surge of insulin to bring down the blood sugar. This extra insulin stimulates oil-producing hormones and accelerates cell growth in the pores, which can lead to acne. That isn't news to Elson Haas, MD, author of *Staying Healthy With Nutrition*, who has long maintained that an ongoing battle with acne is a good indication that your diet is too high in sugar. Although an occasional chocolate chip cookie won't do you in, Haas warns that eating excessive amounts of refined sugar not only overstimulates hormones, it also depletes certain vitamins and minerals necessary for healthy skin.

But sugary snacks aren't the only culprit. All high-glycemic carbohydrates appear to affect the development and severity of acne. Yes, cookies, candy, and soda count, but so does white bread, refined pasta, white rice, and potato chips. And watch out for hidden sugar in canned soups and salad dressings.

Dietary fat also plays a role in acne. Although oils are essential for healthy, attractive skin, too much of the wrong fats can throw your complexion out of whack. An overabundance of saturated fat—primarily found in meat—causes the sebaceous glands to go into overdrive, producing more oil than your system can handle. Leukotriene B4, which causes inflammation, has been implicated in the development of acne. Arachidonic acid is the major omega-6 fatty acid in meat, and it is also the precursor of leukotriene B4.

Trans fats, a particularly harmful type of fat found in many processed foods, also trigger inflammation that can contribute to acne. "A healthful diet rich in natural whole foods like vegetables, fruits, whole grains, and beans is the first recommendation for treating acne," says Michael T. Murray, author of the *Encyclopedia of Nutritional Supplements: The Essential Guide for Improving Your Health Naturally*. "Foods containing trans fatty acids, such as milk, milk products, margarine, shortening, and other synthetically hydrogenated vegetable oils, as well as fried foods, must be avoided." But trans fats aren't just bad for your skin. They have also been implicated in heart disease and cancer. They're so dangerous that some cities and states have actually banned trans fats in restaurants.

But not all fat is bad. Omega-3 essential fatty acids help keep skin smooth and soft while dissolving fatty deposits that block pores. They are also necessary to rebuild and produce new skin cells. Omega-3 fatty acids, found in fatty fish, flaxseeds, and some nuts, can block leukotriene B4 and keep a lid on inflammation. As an added bonus, omega-3s can also improve your mood and feelings of well-being. Try adding omega-3s to your diet by eating more fatty fish like salmon, tuna, and halibut. Flaxseeds and flaxseed oil, as well as pumpkin seeds and walnuts, are all tasty ways to increase your consumption of these healthful fats.

Eating plenty of colorful fruits and vegetables, along with whole grains, can also benefit your complexion. These foods are high in zinc and

(continued on page 26)

Got Acne?

A Word About Milk

You probably grew up thinking that milk was wholesome and nutritious. And yes, milk does have its good points. After all, it's a great source of calcium and vitamin D. But if you are prone to acne, steer clear of this dairy staple, unless it is organic milk from cows that have not been injected with growth hormones and antibiotics.

Researchers from the Harvard School of Public Health investigated data from more than 6,000 middle school and high school girls suffering from acne. Results showed that those who drank the most milk were 22 percent more likely to experience severe acne compared with those who drank less than one serving a week. The results were the same when the researchers tested boys of the same age. What is it about milk? The scientists conducting these two studies believe that the hormones and bioactive molecules in cow's milk are likely responsible for making acne worse.

Along with milk, avoid cottage cheese, cream cheese, and ice cream since these have also been linked to acne flare-ups. Better choices include coconut milk or rice milk products. Many of these dairy alternatives also provide a hefty dose of calcium. But to make sure you are getting all the bone-building calcium you need, it's smart to take a high-quality calcium supplement.

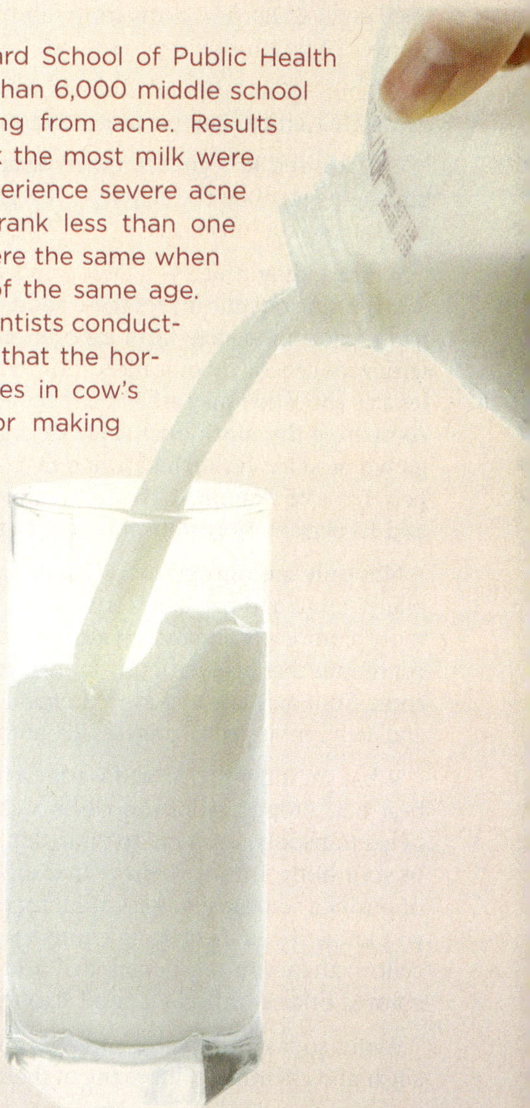

vitamins A, C, and E, nutrients that help prevent the buildup of toxins that can lead to skin problems. They are also bursting with fiber, which is essential for healthy digestion and elimination. Here's where you can find these acne-busting nutrients:

Vitamin A: Found in broccoli, carrots, spinach, cantaloupe, and peaches, vitamin A (as beta-carotene) helps skin resist infection and blemishes.

B-Complex Vitamins: This family of nutrients in whole grains, beans, and legumes reduces oiliness and the formation of blackheads.

Vitamin C: Berries, citrus fruits, and leafy green vegetables are excellent sources of this antioxidant required for tissue growth and repair.

Vitamin E: Can be found in brown rice, soybeans, sweet potatoes, and wheat germ. This antioxidant promotes tissue repair and improves circulation.

Zinc: Found in legumes, mushrooms, soy products, and whole grains, zinc helps regulate the activity of oil glands and promotes more efficient healing of skin infections.

While adding fruits, vegetables, and whole grains to your diet is a good thing, eating organic makes these good foods even better. Not only are certified organic foods free from exposure to pesticides, sewer sludge, synthetic fertilizers, genetic modification, growth hormones, and antibiotics, but studies also show that they are actually more nutritious. In a review of 41 studies comparing the nutritional value of organically grown and conventionally grown produce, researchers found that organic fruits and vegetables offer 27 percent more vitamin C, 21 percent more iron, 29 percent more magnesium, and 13 percent more phosphorus than their conventional counterparts.

Not only are organic foods better for you—they are also better for the planet. Fruits and vegetables grown using sustainable organic techniques promote biodiversity and protect air, soil, and groundwater. Instead of the brutal conditions that plague factory farms, organic meat, eggs, and dairy products come from animals that are fed organic feed, given access to the outdoors, and aren't subjected to unnecessary antibiotics and growth hormones.

What should you drink to wash all this good food down? Water is your best bet. Proper hydration clears waste and toxins from the body and helps transport nutrients to your skin. It also carries oxygen to every cell in your body. I firmly believe that drinking at least eight 8-ounce glasses of purified water daily is essential for good health and clear skin. How do you know if you are getting enough water? Check your urine. If it is dark yellow, then you are dehydrated and need to drink more water. Light-colored or clear urine is a good sign that you are drinking enough.

Avoid sodas and diet drinks. Not only are these beverages a source of sugar and chemicals, but many of them also contain caffeine. Caffeine is a diuretic, and consuming too much can lead to dehydration. Opt instead for herbal teas, especially green tea. Green tea boosts the immune system, reduces inflammation, and speeds up your metabolism, while also balancing the hormones implicated in acne.

Supplements

Although food provides a more balanced and absorbable form of the nutrients needed for a healthy complexion, supplements can play an important role in your clear skin plan. A high-quality multivitamin/mineral is critical, since several deficiencies—including potassium and B vitamins—are associated with acne. Other important vitamins

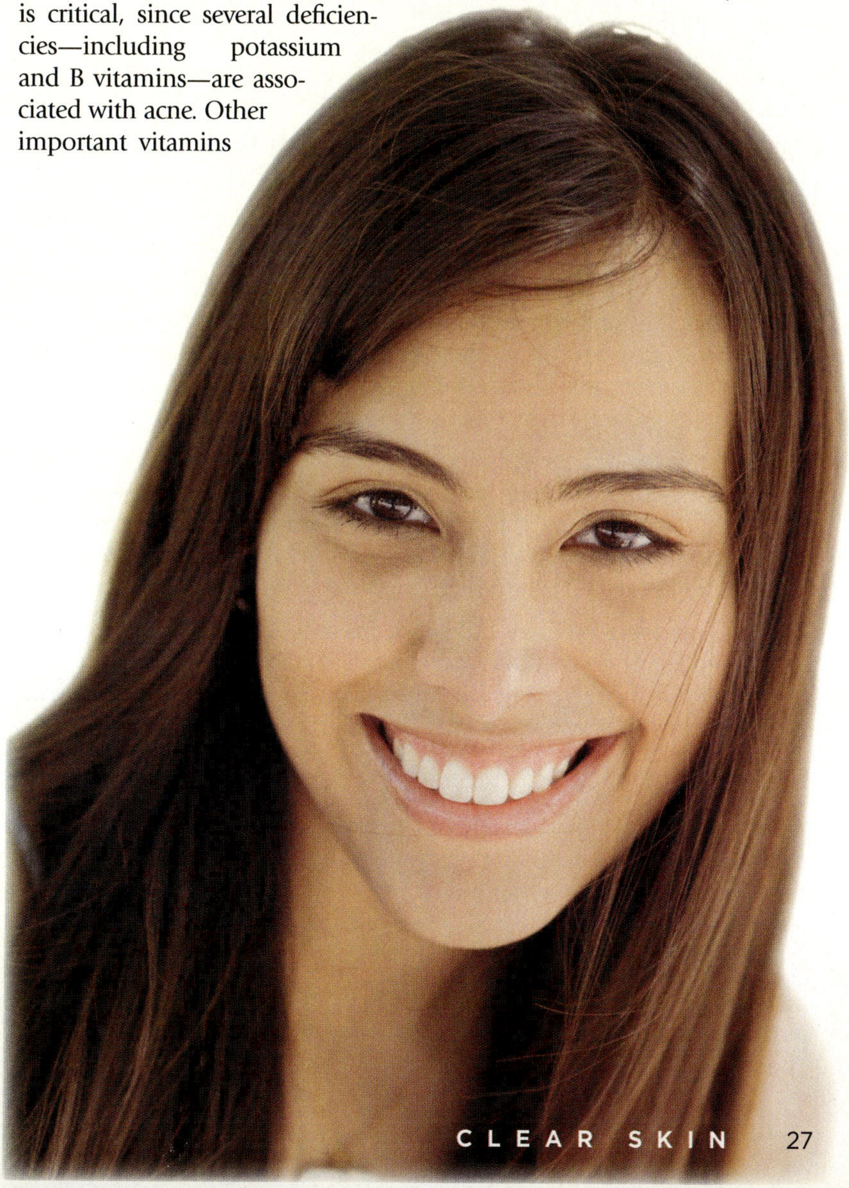

and minerals that help prevent acne eruptions are vitamin A and zinc. Vitamin A is necessary for skin healing. Zinc also aids in healing tissue, helps prevent scarring, and helps the body resist infection and inflammation. One study of zinc and niacinamide (one of the B vitamins) found that combining these two nutrients reduces inflammation, attacks the P. bacteria, and decreases sebum production.

If you don't eat a lot of fish, it's wise to take a separate omega-3 fatty acid supplement. Omega-3 fatty acids have antibacterial and anti-inflammatory effects. They also maintain healthy cell membranes and ensure the normal transport of nutrients into the cells, making omega-3 fats among the most important nutrients for people with acne.

Exercise

It's no secret that daily exercise can be extremely beneficial to your general health. But it can also help clear your skin by increasing the flow of blood and oxygen to the skin cells. Plus, exercise can help your body expel toxins through the skin.

Working out also reduces stress levels and enhances the production of endorphins. Endorphins are chemicals in the brain that promote a sense of well-being and act like natural painkillers. Adopting a regular exercise program also improves both self-image and self-confidence, which can be extremely important for anyone suffering from acne.

While any type of activity is good for you, aerobic exercise boosts circulation and strengthens your immune system. Try walking or jogging for at least 30 minutes daily. If that sounds too mundane for you, mix it up. Biking, soccer, tennis, and swimming are fun ways to boost your cardio. If you can, try to exercise outdoors in the fresh air and sunshine.

When exercising, wear as little makeup as possible. Even oil-free and noncomedogenic cosmetics can clog pores if worn during heavy exercise. When you're done exercising, shower as soon as possible to wash away the sweat and any other waste material purged from the body.

Relaxation

Have you noticed that stress seems to trigger pimples? Well, it isn't just a coincidence. Recent investigations showed that when 94 high school students became stressed while preparing for midterm exams, the quantity of sebum production increased. Stress also has a negative impact on your immune system, slowing the healing process.

Of course, you can't eliminate all stress from your life—it's part of being human. But you can minimize its damage with relaxation techniques. There are all sorts of ways to relieve stress and anxiety: Yoga, meditation, massage, and breath work are proven to calm your mind. But I've found that even something as simple as taking a walk or listening to soothing music eases stress.

The simplest thing you can do to foster a healthy mind and body is to get enough sleep. Scientists and mothers around the world agree that a good night's sleep—between seven and eight hours—can do wonders for your complexion. How? A healthy, well-rested body has the resources to build a strong immune system. While a robust immune system won't prevent acne altogether, it can help fight infection, so your lesions clear up more quickly.

Bad Habits And Breakouts

By now, you've probably realized that adopting healthy habits can have a big impact on both your health and the appearance of your skin. But there are a couple very dangerous habits that can cause acne or make existing acne worse: smoking and anabolic steroid use. Unfortunately, a growing number of teens and young adults are experimenting with both.

It's no secret that cigarette smoking can lead to cancer, stroke, and heart disease. It's also extremely addictive. But did you know that smoking can give you acne? I'm really not surprised. Cigarette smoke contains more than 4,000 toxic chemicals, many of which are absorbed directly into the bloodstream and are taken by the blood right into the structure of your skin.

Smokers can also develop noninflamed blackheads and blocked pores—a condition known as "smoker's acne."

Smoking causes premature wrinkles, especially deep wrinkles around your mouth, cheeks, and chin. It also reduces the efficiency with which the skin can regenerate itself. Smoking constricts (narrows) the blood vessels at the top layers of the skin, which in turn reduces blood supply to the skin. This reduced blood supply decreases the availability of oxygen and hampers the removal of waste products and dead skin cells.

Smokers can also develop noninflamed blackheads and blocked pores—a condition known as "smoker's acne." According to a study by researchers at the San Gallicano Dermatological Institute in Rome, Italy, 42 percent of the smokers involved in the study suffered from acne, compared to just 10 percent of the nonsmokers tested. And when it came to the severity of the acne, it didn't seem to matter how many cigarettes the subjects smoked. Those who only smoked a few cigarettes per day had breakouts that were just as bad as those who smoked a pack or more. The women in the study who smoked were also four times more likely to experience smoker's acne as an adult if they suffered from breakouts during their teen years.

Anabolic steroid use is another problem, not only among professional athletes, bodybuilders, and celebrities, but also among teens. While steroids might seem like a shortcut to better athletic performance, even short-term use can cause liver tumors, jaundice, fluid retention, high blood pressure, heart attacks, reproductive problems, and potentially dangerous psychological changes. But besides these health-threatening side effects, acne occurs in about half of all people who use anabolic steroids. And I'm not talking about the occasional pimple. Many people who abuse steroids find they suffer from severe acne that can lead to scarring. Fortunately, most of the adverse effects of steroid abuse, including acne, are reversible once the drugs are no longer taken.

Anabolic steroids stimulate the production of oil in the skin. Drugs prescribed to treat acne (such as tetracycline and Accutane) may become toxic at normal doses if taken by a steroid abuser. When the liver enzymes are busy detoxifying the steroids, they can't deactivate these prescription drugs at a normal rate. The prescription drugs accumulate in the body, leading to toxic effects.

The short-term gains from using anabolic steroids aren't worth these potentially deadly and disfiguring side effects. Instead of cheating, take the time and do the work required to improve your physical performance. Not only will you be amazed at what you can accomplish, you will also be laying the foundation for lifelong health.

Final Thoughts

I know how agonizing the battle against acne can be—both physically and emotionally. At times it seems like you'll never have clear skin, no matter what you try. But I can also tell you from my own experience that you can overcome acne.

Adopting a daily skin care routine based on effective, pure products that target the underlying causes of acne is the first step toward an acne-free future. If you combine this with a healthy diet, plenty of exercise, and a positive mental outlook, you'll not only begin to discover how terrific you are on the outside, but how wonderful your inside is too. Just remember, good things—including a clear, healthy complexion—take time. Be patient and consistent in caring for your skin, and you will certainly be rewarded with a reflection you will love!

Selected References

Adebamowo CA. Milk consumption and acne in adolescent girls. *Dermatology Online Journal* 12:1, 2006.

Adebamowo CA. Milk consumption and acne in teenage boys. *Journal of the American Academy of Dermatology* 58:787-93, 2008.

Albach DC. Piecing together the "new" Plantaginaceae. *American Journal of Botany* 92:297-315, 2005.

Allmyr M. Triclosan in plasma and milk from Swedish nursing mothers and their exposure via personal care products. *The Science of the Total Environment* 372:87-93, 2002.

Azoulay L. Isotretinoin and the risk of depression in patients with acne vulgaris: a case-crossover study. *The Journal of Clinical Psychiatry* 69:526-632, 2008.

Ballanger F. Heredity: a prognostic factor for acne. *Dermatology* 212:145-9, 2006.

Berard A. Isotretinoin, pregnancies, abortions and birth defects: a population-based perspective. *British Journal of Clinical Pharmacology* 63:196-205, 2007.

Capitanio B. 'Smoker's acne': a new clinical entity? *British Journal of Dermatology* 157:1070-1, 2007.

Evans GB. The synthesis and antibacterial activity of totarol derivatives. Part 3: Modification of ring-B. *Bioorganic and Medicinal Chemistry* 8:1663-75, 2000.

Final Report on the Safety Assessment of Polyvinylpyrrolidone/Vinyl Acetate Copolymer. *International Journal of Toxicology* 2:141-59, 1983.

Fivenson DP. The mechanisms of action of nicotinamide and zinc in inflammatory skin disease. *Cutis* 77:5-10, 2006.

Ganguli S. Neem: A therapeutic for all seasons. *Current Science* 82:1304, 2002.

Garner SE. Minocycline for acne vulgaris: efficacy and safety. *Cochrane Database System Review* CD002086, 2003.

Goulden V. Guidelines for the management of acne vulgaris in adolescents. *Paediatric Drugs* 5:301-13, 2003.

Gupta A. A poly-herbal formulation accelerates normal and impaired diabetic wound healing. *Wound Repair and Regeneration* 16:784-90, 2008.

Gupta AK. The use of sulfur in dermatology. *Journal of Drugs in Dermatology* 3:427-31, 2004.

Györéné KG. A comparison of chemical composition and nutritional value of organically and conventionally grown plant derived foods. *Orvosi Hetilap* 147:2081-90, 2006.

Haas E. *Staying Healthy With Nutrition, 21st Century Edition: The Complete Guide to Diet & Nutritional Medicine*. Berkeley, CA: Celestial Arts, 2006.

Hazlewood C. Benzoyl peroxide-induced damage to DNA and its components: direct evidence for the generation of base adducts, sugar radicals, and strand breaks. *Archives of Biochemistry and Biophysiology* 332:79-91, 1996.

James K. *The Truth About Beauty*. Hillsboro, OR: Beyond Words Publishing, 2007.

Knowles SR. Serious adverse reactions induced by minocycline. Report of 13 patients and review of the literature. *Archives of Dermatology* 32:934-9, 1996.

Liao S. The medicinal action of androgens and green tea epigallocatechin gallate. *Hong Kong Medical Journal* 7:369-74, 2001.

Melnik B. Abuse of anabolic-androgenic steroids and bodybuilding acne: an underestimated health problem. *Journal of the German society of Dermatology* 5:110-7, 2007.

Michalak-Stoma A. The effect of Propionibacterium acnes on maturation of dendritic cells derived from acne patients' peripheral blood mononuclear cells. *Folia Histochemica Cytobiologica* 46:535-9, 2008.

Mills OH. Comparing 2.5%, 5%, and 10% benzoyl peroxide on inflammatory acne vulgaris. *International Journal of Dermatology* 25:664-7, 1984.

Mishell DR. YAZ and the novel progestin drospirenone. *The Journal of Reproductive Medicine* 53:721-8, 2008.

Murray MT. *Encyclopedia of Nutritional Supplements: The Essential Guide for Improving Your Health Naturally* New York, NY: Three Rivers Press, 1996.

Nakamura Y. A phase II detoxification enzyme inducer from lemongrass: identification of citral and involvement of electrophilic reaction in the enzyme induction. *Biochemical and Biophysical Research Communications* 302:593-600, 2003.

Omega-3 Fatty Acids and Acne. *American Academy of Anti-Aging Medicine*, 2004.

Riley M. *Maori Healing and Herbal: New Zealand Ethnobotanical Sourcebook*. Paraparaumu, New Zealand: Viking Seven Seas, 1994.

Rubin MG. Acne vulgaris, mental health and omega-3 fatty acids: a report of cases. *Lipids in Health and Disease* 7:36, 2008.

Smith R. A low-glycemic-load diet improves symptoms in acne vulgaris patients: a randomized controlled trial. *American Journal of Clinical Nutrition* 86:107-15, 2007.

Tan HH. Topical antibacterial treatments for acne vulgaris: comparative review and guide to selection. *American Journal of Clinical Dermatology* 5:79-84, 2004.

Thomas DR. Psychosocial effects of acne. *Journal of Cutaneous Medicine and Surgery* 8S:3-5, 2004.

Tom WL. New insights into adolescent acne. *Current Opinions in Pediatrics* 20:436-40, 2008.

Winter R. *A Consumer's Dictionary of Cosmetic Ingredients*. New York, NY: Three Rivers Press, 2005.

Yosipovitch G. Study of psychological stress, sebum production and acne vulgaris in adolescents. *Acta Dermato Venereologica* 87:135-9, 2007.

Website for Acne Resource

http://www.acne-resource.org/understanding-acne/acne-statistics.html

Website for the Environmental Protection Agency

http://www.epa.gov

Website for the Food and Drug Administration

http://www.fed.gov

Website for the Skin Deep Database, Environmental Working Group

http://www.cosmeticsdatabase.com/

For more information about the products mentioned in this booklet visit:

www.mychelleusa.com